Food for Mood

A guide to healthy eating for mental health

TIM WATKINS
For
LIFE SURFING

Life Surfing

ISBN-13: 978-1492700463
ISBN-10: 1492700460

CONTENTS

Life Surfing

Foreword

Healthy eating can improve your health and sense of wellbeing. Many illnesses are caused or triggered by a shortage of vitamins and minerals.

Most people know that scurvy is caused by a shortage of Vitamin C, and that skeletal problems can result from a shortage of calcium. Perhaps less well known is the effect of tryptophan shortage on people predisposed to depression - clinical trials have shown that when these people are given chemicals that artificially block tryptophan, they quickly experience the onset of depression. Deficiencies of other minerals such as folic acid are also thought to bring on symptoms of depression, but the evidence is less solid.

When it comes to human biology, excess and deficiency can be equally bad. Balance is more often the goal to aim for.

Linus Pauling, a Nobel Laureate in Chemistry drew the logically flawed conclusion that if Vitamin C deficiency is bad for you, then an excess of Vitamin C must be really good for you. In fact, eat too much Vitamin C and your body simply expels the excess. But the same logical flaw persists with other vitamins and minerals, where harm can result. Eat too much Vitamin E and your body will store it in fat, where it will eventually start to poison you (it is unlikely that you would die from this, but it would make you feel unwell). Take too much Tryptophan, or take it alongside SSRI antidepressants and you risk Serotonin poisoning.

The problem is that health food is big business. The supermarkets are full of "healthy eating" products that may be significantly less healthy than food that you can easily and cheaply prepare and cook for yourself. Similarly, health food shops are filled with unnecessary (unless you have a health condition that requires additional intake) and expensive supplements offering vitamins and minerals that are best digested from fresh food (the global nutritional supplement market is worth in excess of $56bn a year).

Rather than worrying unduly about which foods may improve your mental health, you are better off beginning by eating a balanced and varied diet that is low in fat and high in fibre.

I am not going to labour the information about what a balanced diet looks like, because I believe most people already know. Instead, I am going to set out the barriers facing people with mental health problems who wish to eat a healthy balanced diet. I will also indicate some of the ways that these barriers can be overcome.

I have provided some model recipes for fast but healthy foods. Importantly, these are meals that can be ready within 30 minutes, require few saucepans, and do not need much talent for cookery to prepare. The idea is that if you try these out, you will find that cooking from fresh ingredients is a lot easier than you might have been led to believe.

I can't promise that healthy eating will bring about recovery, although I am sure it will improve your general wellbeing. What I can say is that a large number of people who recover also have better diets. And I can promise you that healthy eating will not hurt you. So, give it a try!

Life Surfing

Myths and Messages

You will almost certainly have heard that our diet is in serious decline. You may have heard that the increase in conditions such as cancer, depression, diabetes, heart disease, obesity and strokes results from this deterioration in diet.

Stories based around these two propositions appear every day in newspapers and magazines, and are posted all over the Internet. And they are myths!

However, the "white noise" generated serves to drown out sensible advice about eating, and plays into the hands of a growing "health food" industry that turns over millions of pounds a year from the sale of unnecessary and potentially dangerous food and vitamin supplements every year.

What do we know about diet?

Diet is something we know a lot about. Since 1940 (the year of the Battle of Britain, the Blitz and the start of the U-Boat blockade of Britain) - when the UK really did have a food emergency – the UK government has been keeping detailed records of food intake.

What this annual *National Food Survey* shows is that the British diet has been improving year on year. We eat 1,000 calories less than our grandparents did back in the 1950s. We eat considerably less fat than our parents and grandparents, and the fat that we do eat is much more likely to be unsaturated whereas our grandparents ate unhealthy, saturated fats.

It is true that we eat fewer vegetables than was the case in the 1940s. However, we are eating smaller amounts of a wider range of vegetables than our grandparents did. Moreover, the varieties of fruit that we now eat more than makes up for lower vegetable consumption.

Fish consumption is down, but the fall came in the late 1940s, when Britain's reliance on fish as a source of protein began to fall as imports of fresh meat began to rise. Once again, a more varied diet has replaced reliance on a small range of foods in wartime.

Income can be a factor in diet. In general, the wealthier you are, the healthier your diet will be. However, even people in the lowest income groups can enjoy a healthier diet today than ever before. There is, however, an important exception to this. People living on pensions and benefits tend to eat more unhealthy foods - fats, sugar and preserves, salt, etc - than people in work. There is also a group of people not in work but not on the lowest incomes either, who also eat large amounts of unhealthy foods.

Importantly, people in these groups do eat at least the minimum recommended amounts of healthy foods: they just over-indulge in unhealthy foods too.

What this suggests is that economic inactivity is more of an indicator of unhealthy diet than low income. We can only speculate as to why this should be. However, it seems reasonable to suggest that someone who is active is more likely to stick to regular meal times where someone who is at home for long periods may "comfort eat" between or instead of meals.

So what about illnesses like cancer, depression, diabetes, heart disease, obesity and strokes?

It is one thing to say that what we eat (or don't eat) has a role in disease. It is something quite different to say that our diet is a cause of disease. There are several reasons to be sceptical about claims that illness is caused by diet:

- o Recognition and diagnosis are much improved since the 1940s, so even where there is an increase, the statistics may over-exaggerate it
- o Diet is only one of a number of factors likely to result in illness, others include:
    - o Genes
    - o Physiology
    - o Psychology
    - o Upbringing
    - o Socio-economic circumstances
- o Our best evidence is for the role of food deficiencies in illness (e.g., lack of vitamin C

resulting in scurvy). Evidence that particular foods cause particular illnesses is much weaker

o Much of the obesity that is meant to be a trigger for illness is the result of sedentary lifestyles, not diet. The problem is not food intake but a lack of physical activity to burn excess calories

o Some of those who make the link between diet and illness most vociferously stand to benefit financially from it through the sales of food supplements and health food products.

In something as complex as mental illness, the best we can say is that poor diet is sometimes associated with illness. We cannot say that it is a cause. Nor can we be certain that it is a causal factor. Similarly, we can say that good diet is sometimes associated with recovery. But this is a long way from proof of a therapeutic benefit. It is at least as likely that a deteriorating diet is the result of the onset of illness (especially where illness leads to economic inactivity), while improvements in diet result from improvement in health (particularly where the individual reengages in meaningful social and economic activity).

So where does this leave someone who is concerned about their mental health?

Despite our lack of knowledge about the role of diet in mental health, it is still important to eat a varied and balanced diet in order to promote and sustain a general standard of health and sense of wellbeing: A good diet isn't going to hurt you; a poor diet might.

There is a large body of anecdotal evidence to suggest that some foods when used as part of a balanced diet may promote improved mood and a sense of wellbeing. Although there is no hard evidence to prove this to be true, as with many other elements of recovery, if it works for you, keep doing it!

What is a balanced diet?

Broadly, a balanced diet is based around complex carbohydrates like potatoes, grains and cereals, with plenty of fruit, vegetables and pulses coupled to smaller amounts of protein (e.g. lean meat, fish or eggs). Your diet should ideally be high in fibre and low in salt, sugar and saturated fats.

What is a varied diet?

In addition to balance, the more varied your diet, the healthier it will be. This means not relying on the same foods week-in, week-out. Switching your carbohydrates, fruits and vegetables and sources of protein is the best way of ensuring that you are getting your full complement of vitamins and minerals.

Does it matter if I eat junk food?

There are those who say that, "there is no such thing as junk food - only junk diets". What they mean is that there is nothing wrong with a moderate amount of foods such as chips, ice cream or chocolate.

It is only when these foods become the main part of most meals that problems arise. Too much of these foods can lower your mood and sense of wellbeing, and may result in serious illness in the long term. This is particularly true if you are not physically active enough to use up the energy contained in these foods. In the end, you have to balance your intake of fatty and sugary foods against the amount of energy you burn in your work and recreation.

Unless you are unfortunate enough to have allergies or a health condition that prevents you eating certain foods (in which case your doctor or dietician will be advising you about diet anyway), what you need to know about diet can be written on the back of an envelope.

So, to paraphrase your granny, "eat your greens!"

Mental Illness and Poor Diet

While much attention has been given to the possibility that poor diet may cause mental health problems, less has been given to the ways in which mental health problems may cause poor diet. This is important because broad health messages may well miss the point if they fail to take on board the reasons why someone is not eating healthily. For example, simply telling people to "eat five-a-day" may amount to torture for someone so agoraphobic that they cannot leave the house, let alone shop several times a week for fresh fruit and vegetables.

Understanding and overcoming the barriers to healthy eating are much more important than just offering information.

Poor mental health can affect diet in several different ways:

- o Quick-fix/Comfort eating
- o Anxiety/Agoraphobia
- o Loss of appetite
- o Low motivation
- o Side-effects of medication
- o Imposed socio-economic circumstances

Quick-fix/Comfort eating

Chemicals such as adrenaline and cortisol that are produced within the body when you are under stress are extremely toxic (the amounts produced are so small that you couldn't see them with the naked eye). While the body can eliminate these chemicals from the body over time, there are several substances that can provide short-term relief from the effects of these chemicals. The most common are:

- Alcohol
- Caffeine
- Chocolate
- Nicotine
- Sugar

Smokers are usually aware that when they are stressed they smoke more. They are less likely to notice that smoking increases stress. Many of us will have had alcoholic beverages as an aid to unwinding at the end of a stressful day. Chocolate and sugary food can also mitigate the unpleasant side-effects of stress.

In the short-term, with the exception of smoking, these substances are not a problem. Difficulties arise because each of the substances is addictive. When the stress is prolonged, you need ever-higher doses of these substances to overcome its effects. However, over time, the substances themselves produce unpleasant side effects that serve to add to stress. The danger is that you can get locked into this kind of "self-medicating" behaviour in a way that damages your long-term health.

In addition, the act of eating is pleasurable. For some people binge eating provides a sense of relief that is difficult to resist. There may also be particular psychological associations between certain foods (e.g., chocolate, ice cream, etc) and feeling good. This can result in binge eating when you feel bad, or when you are bored.

Anxiety/Agoraphobia

Extreme fear and distress are common features of mental illness, and can result in withdrawal from day to day activities. Two arenas that are particularly difficult for people affected by anxiety are using public transport and shopping in supermarkets or crowded high streets.

Because healthy food is often also perishable food, a healthy diet may involve several shopping trips every week. For someone experiencing increasing levels of anxiety, this operates as a deterrent. The preference will be for buying non-perishable processed foods (as these will last longer) and sugary foods as these offer an instant energy hit. As such, an anxious person may know what a healthy diet involves, but their anxiety acts to deny them access.

Loss of appetite

Typically, people affected by common mental health problems will lose their appetite. Many will report food seeming tasteless and un-enjoyable. This can result in people eating less and skipping meals. It can also result in people turning to unhealthy processed foods that have added flavour-enhancing chemicals. It may also result in binge eating if high-sugar or high-carbohydrate foods are used as an energy-fix to overcome the hunger resulting from under-eating.

Low motivation

Mental health problems are associated with a lowering of enthusiasm for a range of activities, even those that previously gave great pleasure. This lowering of motivation can make the process of buying, preparing and cooking fresh food too much of a chore.

The combination of lost appetite and low motivation can leave people much more likely to opt for a diet of processed ready meals that are often high in fat, sugar and salt.

Side-effects of medication

In addition to mental health problems themselves, the treatments can impair people's diets. For example, some medications can produce constipation, while SSRI antidepressants like Prozac have been associated with carbohydrate cravings.

Medication may affect taste (this can also be an effect of depression), resulting in a desire for foods that are saltier or more sugary than you would ordinarily want to eat. Also, some people find that sugary food can mitigate some of the side effects associated with medication.

Imposed socio-economic circumstances

The process of becoming ill involves a slide into what has been termed the "sick role". This involves the gradual withdrawal from employment and a consequent lowering of income.

As we have seen, people who are economically inactive have the worse diet of all. And someone who is off work but still receiving sick pay would fall into the group that not only has the desire to over-eat, but also the income to indulge this desire.

The eventual drop in income that results first from going onto half-pay, and eventually moving onto benefits may not be sufficient to overturn eating patterns established during the period of (relatively) high-income economic inactivity. However, it may well impact upon people's ability to access healthy food, for example by limiting their car use and thereby their access to supermarkets.

Maintaining a healthy diet in the face of depression is, then, an uphill struggle. The factors outlined above are seldom experienced in isolation. Most often you will experience a combination of most or all of these factors working against your need to eat healthily.

It should come as no surprise that healthy eating is a battle that many of us lose. And while the resulting poor diet is an effect of the condition rather than a cause, it may well become one of a range of factors that stands in the way of recovery. As such, it is important to try to overcome the barriers to healthy eating associated with mental illness as part of an overall approach to recovery.

Food Poverty

Even if you are able to overcome the barriers to healthy eating created by your mental illness, there are additional societal barriers that must also be overcome. Collectively, these barriers have been termed "food poverty".

Although much of the official concern about food poverty has focused on the barriers facing older people, there is a growing recognition that a much wider population - including people with physical and mental illnesses - may be affected.

Food poverty is defined as an inability to maintain a healthy diet due to issues around:

- o   Accessibility
- o   Availability
- o   Affordability
- o   Awareness

Accessibility

Most of the literature on food poverty focuses on changes in patterns of food retailing and public transport in recent decades.

The decline of high street shopping, the growth of car ownership and the development of large, out-of-town supermarkets may have allowed for improved choice and convenience for the affluent, but for groups like those on benefits, these developments have meant a lack of access.

Disability adds another dimension to accessibility. By installing disabled parking, ramped access, sliding doors, etc, most large retailers are able to meet the needs of people with physical disabilities. However, for people with mental health problems, access is more about the psychological distress involved in using large, bright, crowded stores. Supermarkets (along with public transport) are the most commonly cited places where panic attacks occur.

Simply knowing a panic attack is likely may be enough to deter someone with mental health problems from making the trip.

Availability

Healthy foods are generally more perishable than processed foods. They also have less "added value", and therefore less of a profit margin. The result is that smaller retailers are reluctant to stock them, while larger retailers need to know that foods will be bought, and not left to go off on the shelf.

Even big supermarkets tend to follow rather that lead demand in stocking healthy food. This means that in areas where bad diet has prevailed across generations, demand for healthy foods will not be as strong, and supermarkets will tend not to over-stock these foods.

Affordability

There is a myth that healthy eating is expensive eating. The large number of processed foods that are labelled as being "healthy", together with the plethora of supplements and additives fuels this belief. However, the healthiest foods come without any packaging at all - fruit, vegetables, potatoes, grains, etc.

It is true that these can be expensive when bought from supermarkets, where value has been added through cleaning, chopping and packaging. Also, supermarkets make a point of accessing fruit and vegetables from around the world so that they are available all year round. However, locally sourced fruit and vegetables that are in season will be cheaper (a strawberry flown in from the other side of the world in mid-winter is going to be more expensive than a local strawberry on sale in the summer).

Supermarkets are not the only retailers in town. Local markets, local box schemes (delivered to your door), green grocers, barrows, green gym allotments and pick-your-own can offer fruit and vegetables that are as healthy at a lower price. This is because:

o They are more likely to be in-season
o They are more likely to be locally grown
o They will require washing and preparing
o They may be misshapen and/or have skin blemishes, so that even though there is nothing

wrong with them, a supermarket will reject them for aesthetic reasons.

Fresh fruit and vegetables can be frozen, so with management it is possible to buy food when it is cheap in order to eat it at a later date.

Awareness

Most of us are aware of the headline messages about healthy eating, such as:

- o Eat less salt
- o Eat less sugar
- o Eat more fibre
- o Eat less fat
- o Eat at least 5 portions of fruit and vegetables every day.

The likelihood is that what you think you know about healthy eating is correct. It is simply that the huge number of features and articles about food and the vast array of specialist diets serve to mystify the whole subject. So as a broad guide:

- o Food that is fresh and unpackaged (or food frozen when fresh) is best
- o Supplements, detox agents and health food products are unnecessary and could be dangerous
- o Specialist diets seldom work even for weight loss

o   Food that has been processed isn't necessarily unhealthy, but you should check the labelling for sugar, salt and fat content

Many manufacturers and retailers operate a traffic light scheme in which healthy food is given a green light, and unhealthy food is given a red light. This means that food with a green light can be eaten as often as you like, food with an amber light can be eaten in moderation, and food with a red light should be eaten sparingly.

Despite a sense of mistrust of government in relation to health, official websites such as the Food Standards Agency (www.food.gov.uk, Helpline: 07823 445801) provide the best available source of advice on diet.

Awareness also includes knowledge about how to prepare and serve healthy food. With cooking and home economics removed from the school curriculum, more and more children are leaving school with little idea where to purchase healthy food or how to prepare and serve it. This can leave you reliant on processed foods that are less likely to be healthy than those cooked from fresh ingredients.

Life Surfing

Overcoming Barriers

If simply telling people to "eat 5-a-day" were sufficient, we would all be eating healthily. We are not.

Most of us understand why healthy eating is important, and have a good idea of what a healthy diet looks like. A few people make a conscious decision not to eat healthily. For most of us, unhealthy diet comes from a range of personal and societal barriers of the kind outlined above.

To try to overcome mental health-related barriers in one go would be setting oneself up to fail. Add to that trying to overcome the societal obstacles to healthy eating and you are almost guaranteed failure.

So does that mean that people with mental health problems should simply resign themselves to an unhealthy diet? Far from it! The trick is to break the tasks facing you into small, manageable steps and to plan ahead.

Coping with the immediate barriers

In the short term, it is more important that you eat well than it is that you overcome your mental health problem. So tackling access issues will be the first problem to overcome.

If you are unable to shop for fresh food either because of agoraphobia or because of transport problems, you need to find a way to bring the food to you.

If you have an Internet connection, this may be less of a problem as, for a small charge, several large food retailers deliver shopping door-to-door. So an immediate solution could be to purchase food online.

Of course, there are difficulties with this. Not everyone has an Internet connection, and not everyone who can log on to a major retailer's website will be able to purchase goods - some retailers refuse to accept payments from people with basic bank accounts.

You should also be aware that this solution will do nothing to help overcome your agoraphobia, and may even make it worse by promoting further social withdrawal.

If Internet shopping is not an option, then it may be that you have to find a way of getting someone else to do your shopping for you. The easiest way will be to secure the help of a relative or friend who is prepared to pick up food for you. However, not everyone is fortunate to have this option.

Other options for getting food to people have been developed, although this varies from area to area. In some areas there will be voluntary sector "food trains", where volunteers take orders from older and disabled people in the community, then pick up and deliver food door-to-door. Understandably, the stigma around mental illness may deter people from identifying themselves to the providers of such schemes. As it is long-term health that is on the line, a balance has to be struck between the benefits of eating healthily and the perceived negative consequences of stigma.

People who qualify for support from social services may also be able to secure support with shopping. However, this type of support is seldom available to people with mental health problems.

These immediate solutions may create further problems as they tend to inhibit recovery from the mental health problems that may be the primary reason behind an unhealthy diet. For example, using the Internet to avoid the anxiety associated with using public transport and/or shopping in a big supermarket or town centre may well reinforce the underlying agoraphobia, making it even more difficult to face these barriers later on.

The long-term goal must be to reach a point where you are able to use public transport and shop in a supermarket or a large town centre.

Dealing with anxiety

There is no "one best way" of dealing with anxiety. However, as a general rule, avoiding a situation tends to reinforce the anxiety while facing it helps overcome the anxiety. The problem is that if you try to face your fears too quickly, this can result in so negative and distressing an experience that this too reinforces the anxiety.

Tackling anxiety in small steps may offer the best results. If for example, a relative or friend has been getting shopping for you, what about asking them to help you go shopping for yourself. This might need to involve several steps over time. For example:

- They accompany you to a small shop where you buy 4 or 5 key items such as bread and eggs
- They wait in the car while you go into a small shop and buy 4 or 5 key items
- They accompany you to a small supermarket where you buy 7 or 8 key items
- They wait in the car while you go into a small supermarket where you buy 7 or 8 key items
- They accompany you to a large supermarket where you buy 9 or 10 key items
- They wait in the car while you go into a large supermarket where you buy 9 or 10 key items (and use the express check out)
- They accompany you while you do a large shop at a large supermarket
- They wait in the car while you do a large shop at a large supermarket

The number of steps will vary from individual to individual. Someone who is very agoraphobic may need several additional intermediate steps, while someone who is anxious but not agoraphobic may be able to miss out a few steps.

Overcoming the anxieties and phobias that often accompany mental health problems is a key element in recovery. Someone who has recovered would be expected to be able to use public transport and shop for food without difficulty. However, this will not necessarily happen overnight.

Life Surfing

Shopping on a budget

It is easy to think that a healthy diet is an expensive diet. If you buy food from an expensive supermarket located miles from your home, this may be true - particularly if you enjoy out of season fruits and vegetables and if you purchase lots of processed foods.

The big supermarkets buy top grade produce. They will reject food that is misshapen and/or blemished. They will also 'add value' to these products by washing, chopping and packaging them - i.e., doing things for an additional price that we are all able to do at home.

The food industry also adds (economic) value to food by processing and packaging it on our behalf. For a price, we get an instant meal and the industry makes a profit.

Supermarket shopping

Supermarkets can be a good source of bargains, but they employ many devices to persuade you to buy more expensive produce while you are shopping. If you are shopping on a budget, you need to stick firmly to the products on your shopping list and not be diverted into impulse buying.

It is a good idea not to take children shopping as many retailers use 'pester pressure' - advertising aimed at children who, in turn pester their parents into buying - to get you to spend more. It is also sensible not to shop on an empty stomach, as this can result in your buying more food than you had intended.

Remember that bargains are only bargains if you set out to buy them. You haven't really got a bargain if you bought something you didn't want for half price - you have still paid more than you intended.

Look out for end of sell-by-date produce. Supermarkets will slash the prices of durable goods before resorting to throwing them out. If you are shopping for a meal today, or if you are able to freeze food, then buying produce that has almost reached its sell-by-date can save a considerable amount of money.

Try to keep an eye on which foods are in season. These are more likely to have been produced locally and are likely to be cheaper than if they had been flown or shipped in.

One way of avoiding the sales techniques used by the supermarkets is to shop online. Because some supermarket websites allow you to keep a shopping list, it is easy to place the same order week in, week out. So although it may cost you an additional £5 to buy in this way, once you factor in any impulse purchases that you might otherwise have made, and once transport costs have been deducted, you may well be better off.

Markets, grocers and street barrows

If you are prepared to put a bit more effort into preparing food, you are more likely to stay within budget by using markets, grocers and street barrows. These tend not to stock the range of produce available from the supermarkets, largely because they will not have bought as much of the produce that has to be flown or shipped in.

These retailers will buy second grade produce that is fine to eat, but may be misshapen and/or blemished. Unlike the supermarkets, they will not have washed, chopped or packaged the produce - you will have to do this when you get home.

As with the supermarkets, there are bargains to be had as food comes up to its sell-by-date. Spark up a relationship with the local grocer, and find out when and on which days he or she has produce left over, and you may well get it at a significant reduction. Indeed, if you shop with the same grocer most of the time, your personal relationship may make it more likely that you will get a bargain than if you are dealing with the faceless pricing managers in a large supermarket chain.

Markets can also be a source of bargains as they are more likely to offer locally produced and in-season produce. However, these days, not all markets are cheaper than supermarkets. If the goods on sale are expensive to produce, or if they have been shipped from one end of the country to the other, then you may end up paying as much, if not more than you would have paid in the local grocer's.

Food banks

In recent years there has been a big growth in the numbers of people having to call on charity food banks to supplement the small amounts of food they can buy with benefits or low wages.

Although food banks are able to provide free food, greater care needs to be taken in finding healthy foods. Food banks prefer non-perishable and often high-calorie foods such as tinned fruit, jams and tinned puddings. While these are fine as part of a balanced and varied diet, they should not be all that you eat.

You will have a healthier diet if you can supplement the tinned and dried food you receive from a food bank with fresh vegetables and fruit bought elsewhere.

Food co-operatives

In some communities, groups of people may club together to purchase wholesale food. This means cutting out the grocer. The advantage of this is that you can access food at cost price.

However, you still have to wash and chop the food for yourself. You also have to compete with the other food retailers for the best available produce, and this can eat into the reductions that you get from buying wholesale.

You also need to be aware that food cooperatives are not always aimed at keeping costs down in order to help people make the most of a low income. Cooperatives that aim to encourage the purchase of organic foods, or that are designed to support local farmers or whose primary focus is the environment may actually be more expensive than shopping at the local grocers. So don't simply assume that you are going to save money - check before joining.

Life Surfing

What is a healthy diet?

Remember that there is no such thing as junk food, only junk diets. The aim is not to adopt the lifestyle of some self-flagellating puritanical recluse who lives on a diet of raw turnips. Rather, the aim is to have a balanced and varied diet that provides you with the full range of vitamins and minerals needed to ensure health and to promote a sense of wellbeing.

What is a balanced diet?
Unfortunately for those of us who enjoy chocolate, a balanced diet does not mean three bars of chocolate balanced against a portion of carrots. Indeed, the term "balance" is a little misleading, since the ideal is one third complex carbohydrates[1], one third fruit and vegetables, a quarter milk, dairy products, meat and fish (and alternatives such as Quorn), and the remaining 9% for fatty and/or sugary foods.

This is an ideal, and you should not beat yourself up if you do not achieve it. However, the closer you can get to this ideal the better.

What is a varied diet?
In order to obtain the full range of vitamins and minerals, it is important to have as much variety as

---

[1] Complex carbohydrates are starchy foods such as pasta, potatoes, grains and bread. These are broken down in the body to produce glucose. They are a much healthier source of energy than simple carbohydrates like refined sugar.

possible in your diet. This means using a broad range of foods rather than relying on the same foods day in, day out.

One of the myths about people's diets during the Second World War is that people ate healthily because they ate a large quantity of vegetables. However, because much of this intake was from home grown produce that was seasonal, there was a greater reliance on root vegetables such as carrots. Moreover, with other foods in short supply, people were more dependent on staples such as bread and pastry to bulk up meals. Thus, while the Second World War diet was balanced, it lacked variety.

This is in stark contrast to the contemporary diet. While we eat fewer vegetables (and much more fruit) we eat from a greater range - modern transportation coupled to freezing means that our diet is less governed by the seasons.

A varied diet, then, is one where we pick and choose from a broad range of ingredients. This offers the best prospect of avoiding the health consequences of deficiencies in vitamins and minerals.

Is fast food junk food?

There is a common misconception that fast food is bound to be junk food. This is probably because of the association between certain high street convenience food outlets and reconstituted/rendered meat products that are often dripping in saturated fats and lacking in fibre. Over time, this view of fast food has spilled over to encompass almost anything that can be served quickly.

This is a particular problem in relation to microwave ready meals that may or may not be healthy. Microwave ovens heat food by "exciting" the water molecules within the food. They do not alter the composition of the food, nor do they irradiate it. Indeed, in terms of preserving the nutrients, food cooked in a microwave oven is likely to be better for you than food boiled in a saucepan.

Ready meals are no more or less healthy than any other cooked meal. It all depends on whether the ingredients are high in fibre and low in fat, salt and sugar. It will also depend on how many steps removed the meal is from the raw ingredients.

The degree to which something is recognisably made from raw ingredients is best determined by looking. That is, if you see vegetables or pieces of lean meat, this is likely to be better than if you see puree and/or pastry.

Judging fat, salt and sugar content is a little trickier. Government and the Food Standards Agency are encouraging a traffic light system of food labelling that uses a red light for foods that are high in fat/salt/sugar, an amber light for foods that are medium and a green light for foods that are low.

Unfortunately, not all manufacturers and retailers have adopted this approach. Where the traffic light system is not used, you will most likely find a label that gives you the amount of fats, salt and sugar as a percentage of recommended daily intakes.

Nor is microwave food necessarily the fastest food. Fast and healthy meals can also be cooked using a steamer, a pressure cooker, or may be oven-baked. Indeed, it is often no quicker to cook unhealthy food than it is to prepare a healthy meal. Anyone who uses a wok for cooking will tell you that it is quicker to rustle up a stir fry than it is to re-heat a microwave meal. A stir fry made up of lean meat and fresh vegetables and cooked in a small amount of unsaturated oil is a fast and healthy meal.

Substances thought to promote mental health and wellbeing are readily available in the quantities required in the ordinary foods that we eat day in, day out. So long as these foods are used as part of a balanced diet, and not eaten to excess, they are highly unlikely to cause harm, and may serve to promote health.

So rather than simply giving you a list of vitamins and minerals thought to promote mental health and wellbeing, we have provided a list of common foods that contain each substance, so that you can think about including these in your diet - indeed, in many cases, you probably already do.

Good mood foods:

- ✓ Essential fats (omega 3, 6 and 9 - especially omega 3)
- ✓ Foods containing anti-oxidants (vitamins A, C and E, beta carotene and bioflavonoids
- ✓ Selenium
- ✓ B vitamins (especially vitamin B6) and folic acid
- ✓ Magnesium
- ✓ Manganese
- ✓ Potassium
- ✓ Zinc
- ✓ Tryptophan

Remember that these should be included as part of a balanced diet, not as part of a fad-diet that would leave you deficient in other essential vitamins and minerals.

Foods containing essential fats:

- o Almonds
- o Avocado
- o Brazil nuts
- o Cashews
- o Evening primrose oil
- o Hazelnuts
- o Hempseed
- o Macadamia nuts
- o Olives
- o Peanuts
- o Pecans

- Pistachio nuts
- Pumpkin seeds
- Sesame seeds
- Sunflower seeds
- Walnuts
- Wheat germ

Foods high in omega 3:

- Anchovies
- Caviar
- Eels
- Fresh tuna
- Herring
- Mackerel
- Pilchards
- Salmon
- Trout

Foods containing anti-oxidants (vitamins A, C and E, beta carotene and bioflavonoids:

- Almonds
- Avocados
- Beans
- Berries
- Blackcurrants
- Broccoli
- Brussels sprouts
- Cabbage
- Carrots
- Cashew nuts

- Cauliflower
- Citrus fruits
- Dried apricots
- Eggs
- Fish liver oil
- Hazelnuts
- Kiwi fruit
- Liver
- Mangos
- Melon
- Oranges
- Organ meats
- Papaya
- Pumpkin
- Red & green peppers
- Seeds
- Spinach
- Sweet potato
- Tangerines
- Tomatoes
- Vegetable oils
- Walnuts
- Watercress

Foods containing selenium:

- Brazil nuts
- Cabbage
- Chicken
- Courgettes
- Herring

- Seafood
- Sesame seeds
- Sunflower seeds
- Tuna
- Whole grains

Foods containing B vitamins and folic acid:

- Avocados
- Bananas
- Beans
- Carrots
- Eggs
- Fish
- Greens
- Lentils
- Meat
- Milk
- Molasses
- Nuts
- Seeds
- Spinach
- Whole grains
- Yeast

Foods high in vitamin B6:

- Avocados
- Bananas
- Brown rice
- Cabbage
- Carrots

- o Cauliflower
- o Chickpeas
- o Egg Yolk
- o Fish
- o Lentils
- o Oat flakes
- o Organ meat
- o Peanuts
- o Peas
- o Potatoes
- o Poultry
- o Prunes
- o Red kidney beans
- o Red Meat
- o Sunflower seeds
- o Sweet potatoes
- o Walnuts
- o Wheat bran
- o Wheat germ
- o Yeast extract

Foods containing magnesium:
- o Leafy green vegetables
- o Nuts
- o Whole grains

Foods containing manganese:
- o Beetroot
- o Blackberries

- Butter beans
- Celery
- Grapes
- Lettuce
- Oats
- Pineapple
- Raspberries
- Strawberries
- Watercress

Foods containing potassium:

- Almonds
- Apricots
- Avocado
- Bananas
- Beans
- Cabbage
- Cashew nuts
- Cauliflower
- Celery
- Courgettes
- Melon
- Mushrooms
- Parsley
- Pumpkin
- Radishes
- Sunflower seeds
- Watercress

Foods that contain zinc:

- o Brazil nuts
- o Herring
- o Meats (especially lamb)
- o Oysters
- o Pumpkin seeds
- o Sesame seeds
- o Sunflower seeds
- o Walnuts
- o Whole grains

Foods containing tryptophan:

- o Bananas
- o Brazil Nuts
- o Bread
- o Chicken
- o Dates
- o Hazelnuts
- o Turkey

Remember that this list is not exhaustive - there are many other fresh ingredients that contain the vitamins and minerals required for a healthy diet. Also, since many of the foods in the list contain several of the vitamins and minerals listed, there is plenty of scope for including them in everyday recipes.

The burgeoning "nutrition industry[2]" currently favoured by television and newspaper editors, also

---

[2] These are companies that sell food additives and supplements (many of which border on being medicines as a result of the claims

serves to mystify what is, in the end, some very straightforward advice. If you are trying to sell someone fish oil pills, you are not going to tell them that they can get all the omega-3 they need (and a bit of Tryptophan and Vitamin B6 to go with it) by eating sardines on toast!

made on their behalf) rather than promoting healthy eating.

Preparing and Cooking Food

One of the biggest barriers to healthy eating is that we have lost knowledge about food that was common to our grandparents. There are several reasons for this, including:

- o Families no longer sitting together to eat
- o Schools no longer teaching cookery/home economics
- o The growth of convenience foods, and the advertising of these
- o Easier and cheaper access to restaurants (of all kinds).

A lack of knowledge can leave people unnecessarily dependent on processed foods. Although these are not necessarily unhealthy, because they are several steps removed from the raw ingredients, there is a greater likelihood of them containing excess fats, salt and sugar.

Preparing food

There is no point attempting to improve your sense of wellbeing through a healthier diet if you are going to get food poisoning in the process, so it is important that you take reasonable care with the food you buy. Food poisoning can result from chemicals, bacteria and viruses that contaminate food. Although much is done to minimise the risk in the production and retail of food, a risk remains. Unfortunately, there is no easy way of telling whether food is contaminated, so we all have to take some precautions. There is no need to be obsessive about this. Just take a few simple steps:

1. Avoid cross-contamination
2. Store food properly
3. Keep yourself, your cooking utensils and your kitchen clean
4. Rinse your food
5. Cook your food thoroughly

Avoid cross-contamination

One important way of minimising the risk of food poisoning is to prevent any chemicals or germs from spreading from one food to another. This is especially true for meat, fish, eggs and dairy products, which should always be kept separate from each other and from other foods until they are ready to be cooked.

Fresh meat and fish should be stored in sealed containers at the bottom of the fridge so that fluids are unlikely to leak out, and those that do will not drip onto other foods.

When preparing food, containers and surfaces that have been used for preparing meat, fish, eggs and dairy produce should be cleaned before being used for preparing other foods.

Similar care should be taken with the contents of tinned or packaged processed foods if you do not intend using them straight away.

Fresh vegetables and dry foods such as flour and pasta may not need to be refrigerated, but they are best kept in separate containers, which should be cleaned periodically.

Storing food

Most food will go off quite quickly if left at room temperature. This is particularly true for many of the fresh ingredients that this booklet encourages you to use. However, there are things you can do to minimise the danger of eating food that has gone off.

If you are going to buy frozen foods or foods that have to be kept refrigerated, it is worth buying these immediately before you return home, so that they remain cold. If you cannot get them home (and into the fridge or freezer) quickly, consider carrying them in a cold bag, or at least insulate them in paper and put them in a cardboard box.

Consider planning a menu for each week. This will help you decide when you need to shop, and what types of food to buy. If, for example, you are shopping on a Friday for food you will use the following Thursday, frozen and tinned foods will be better than fresh ingredients (unless you intend freezing them).

If you freeze foods, remember they will start to go off again as soon as they thaw. So if you froze some food a day before its sell by date, then you will need to eat it within a day of thawing.

Unless you are going to use a microwave oven to thaw food, it is better to allow it to defrost in the fridge. Although this will take longer, it allows for the food to defrost evenly.

Many foods carry the label "keep refrigerated". These foods do not need to be frozen, but they will quickly go off if left at room temperature. It is important that they are kept in the fridge for most of the time.

Keep yourself, your cooking utensils and your kitchen clean

Keeping clean does not require a huge effort. All you need is a bowl of hot water, some soap and some detergent (or you can use a mix of vinegar, bicarbonate of soda and lemon as a cheap and effective cleaner). If you are someone who worries about germs, you might want to use one of the chemical sprays that claims to kill germs and viruses, but a good detergent and some hot water is all that is really needed to remove any dirt and fat that will harbour germs.

Wash your hands before and after preparing food and between preparing different types of food to avoid cross contamination.

If you use a chopping board for preparing meat or fish – especially a wooden one - make sure it is thoroughly cleaned in boiling (or as close as you can get to boiling) water before it is reused. Using a different chopping board for other types of food is worth considering.

Wiping down surfaces before preparing food is important. The same is true of kitchen utensils, which should be washed after use, and stored in a clean place.

It is especially important to keep things clean when preparing meat, fish, eggs and dairy produce.

Rinse your food
To get rid of any chemicals or germs on the surface of food, give it a rinse under the cold tap. There is no need to use any soap, detergent or chemicals.

Remember that washing alone is no guarantee against germs. Also, running water too hard risks cross-contamination if the spray lands on other food. So whether you wash food or not it is important to cook it thoroughly.

Cooking food

Cook meat, fish and eggs thoroughly
The most important way of avoiding food poisoning is to make sure your food is cooked thoroughly.

Most vegetables and seeds are safe to eat either raw or cooked. Pulses are important exceptions, especially red kidney beans and soya beans. These have to be boiled thoroughly before use in cooking to remove naturally occurring toxins (tinned beans will have already been pre-boiled and are safe to cook). In all cases, it is advisable to read the packaging and follow the instructions carefully.

Fresh meat, fish and eggs are much more likely to harbour germs, so it is important that they are properly cooked, as the cooking temperature will kill germs. To tell whether meat is cooked, pierce at the thickest part with a sharp knife; if there is any blood in the juices that flow when the knife is released, it needs more cooking.

Cooking on a budget

With energy prices rising remorselessly, it is important to be energy efficient when cooking. There are several things to consider in keeping costs down:

- o Cooking on a gas hob can be more efficient (and often as quick) as using a microwave. Since the electricity used to power a microwave is more expensive than the gas used to power a hob, gas cooking will be cheaper even if it takes a little longer.
- o Try to use one- or two-pan recipes.

- o Invest in a pressure cooker – these allow you to boil a range of foods in one pot, and the use of pressure means that foods cook more quickly.
- o Invest in a slow cooker – Once food comes to the boil, the only reason for continuing to heat it is to replace heat that evaporates from the top of the pan. A slow cooker uses a vacuum (similar to a flask) to prevent heat loss. Taking the pan off the hob an sealing it in a slow-cooker allows it to fully cook without the need to use additional fuel.

Life Surfing

Basic Food for Mood Recipes

A final barrier to healthy eating is the commonly held view that cooking is complicated. While TV programmes such as *Ready Steady Cook* have done much to demonstrate the ease with which a meal can be created from basic ingredients in less than 30 minutes, many of us still regard cooking as being beyond our capacity.

One reason for this is that people set their sights too high and end up failing. The more complicated a recipe is, the more likely you are to make a mistake. This is particularly true where a range of ingredients have to be cooked separately for various times with the end goal of having everything perfectly cooked at the same time.

Before trying this type of cooking, it is worth trying out some basic recipes. The recipes set out here are for:

- o Spaghetti Bolognese
- o Curry
- o Chilli
- o Stir fry
- o Fish with parsley sauce
- o Stew

The reasons for giving these recipes are:

- ✓ You can prepare them quickly
- ✓ You can use any ingredients you like
- ✓ You only need one or two pans

- ✓ You can learn to make them to taste through trial and error
- ✓ You can make them with or without meat
- ✓ You can cheat

Equipment

For all of the recipes you will need:

- ✓ A chopping board and a sharp chopping knife
- ✓ A large saucepan
- ✓ A large serving bowl
- ✓ A spatula
- ✓ A table spoon
- ✓ A tin opener
- ✓ A wok or a large frying pan

The recipes are given for 2 people.

Spaghetti Bolognese

(Contains: antioxidants, B vitamins and folic acid, vitamin B6, manganese, potassium, zinc)

Ingredients

1 carrot
1 celery stick
1 clove of garlic
1 onion
100g Pasta
1x 400g tins of plum tomatoes
250g minced beef
Basil (dried)

Oregano (dried)
Parsley (fresh)
Pepper
Tomato Puree

Method

Clean and chop the carrot and the celery into small
chunks. Peel and chop the onion. Peel and crush the
garlic.
Half-fill the saucepan with water and bring to the boil,
then add pasta. Simmer for 10-15 minutes until soft
but firm.

Meanwhile, put about 2 tablespoons of olive oil into the
wok and warm it on a medium heat. Add the chopped
onion and garlic.

When these start to sizzle, add the meat, stirring with
the spatula until cooked (5 to 10 minutes). Stir in the
chopped carrot and celery and continue stirring. Stir in
the tinned tomatoes and bring to the boil.

Add about ½ tube of tomato puree and about a
teaspoon each of basil, oregano. Add pepper to taste.

Simmer for 5-10 minutes.

When ready, strain the pasta, serve it on a plate and
pour over the Bolognese. Add the parsley as a garnish.

Cheats

You can buy tins/jars of pour-over pasta sauces. Simply cook the onion and meat, pour on the sauce, simmer then serve.

You can buy garlic puree to save having to chop and crush garlic cloves.

You can add/substitute chopped vegetables to taste – e.g., instead of chopped carrot and celery, try pouring in a tin of ratatouille.

You don't have to use beef. While using other meat or fish would mean that it isn't strictly a Bolognese sauce, it still makes for a quick and tasty meal.

Chicken Curry

(Contains: selenium, B vitamins and folic acid, vitamin B6, tryptophan, potassium,)

Ingredients

- 1 clove of garlic
- 1 medium sized aubergine
- 1 onion
- 1 potato
- 1 tablespoon of plain natural Yoghurt
- 1 teaspoon of garam masala
- 100g of peas
- 100g of string beans
- 2 small carrots
- 2 tablespoons of chopped coriander

250g chicken strips
250g of white rice
3 medium sized tomatoes
39
4 hot green chillies
50g cup of grated coconut
A handful of white poppy seeds
Olive oil

Method

Place the coconut, chillies and poppy seeds into a bowl. Add 150ml water. Crush/grind into a spice paste (use a blender if you have one). Set to one side.
Chop the tomatoes and set aside.

Chop the onion and garlic.

Place the rice in a saucepan of water, bring to the boil and simmer for 10-15 minutes, until the rice is soft.

Chop the aubergine, carrots and potato into strips about the size of your little finger. Place these, along with the peas and string beans into a saucepan and add 250ml water. Bring to the boil, cover and simmer for 4 minutes.

Put about 2 tablespoons of olive oil in the wok and warm on a medium heat. Add the chopped onion, garlic and the chicken and heat until the chicken is cooked.

Add the cooked chicken and the spice paste and another 150ml of water. Stir and simmer gently for 5 minutes.

Add the tomatoes, yoghurt and garam masala. Stir until well mixed. Bring to the boil and simmer for 2-3 minutes.

Cheats

Instead of making your own spice paste, buy a tube or jar of curry paste. Alternatively, use a pour-over curry sauce.

You can use any meat you like, or simply leave out the meat and have a vegetable curry. And you can add or subtract vegetables according to your personal tastes.

Chilli

(Contains: antioxidants, B vitamins and folic acid, vitamin B6, zinc)

Ingredients

1 400g tin of chopped tomatoes
1 beef stock cube
1 clove of garlic
1 onion
1 stick of cinnamon
1 teaspoon of ground coriander
1 teaspoon of ground cumin
1 tin of red kidney beans
2 glasses of red wine

2 red chillies
2 tablespoons of tomato puree
250g lean minced beef
Olive oil
Pepper
Rice
Worcester sauce

Method

Chop the onion and chop and crush the garlic. Cut the chillies into slices. Drain the kidney beans.

Add 2 tablespoons oil to the wok and warm on a medium heat. Add onion and garlic and cook until they begin to sizzle. Turn up the heat and add the minced beef, stirring to break down any lumps. Pour in the red wine and stir for 2 minutes.

Add rice to a saucepan of water, bring to the boil and gently simmer for 15 minutes so that it is ready alongside the chilli.

Add the tinned tomatoes and stir in the chillies, cumin cinnamon and crumble in the beef stock cube. Simmer for 20 minutes then stir in the kidney beans and coriander.

Add pepper and Worcester sauce according to your taste.

Cheats

Dispense with the red wine, garlic, chillies, cumin, cinnamon, pepper and Worcestershire sauce and buy a pour over sauce instead.

Stir fry vegetables

(Contains: antioxidants, B vitamins and folic acid, vitamin B6, potassium, magnesium, selenium)

Ingredients

1 large carrot

1 red pepper

1 tablespoon of brown sugar

1 tablespoon of rice wine or sherry

1 tablespoon of soy sauce

100g bag of beansprouts

1 ½ teaspoons of cornflour

1 ½ teaspoons of lemon or lime juice

1 ½ teaspoons of sesame oil

4 spring onions

4 string beans

Olive oil

Pepper

Tobasco sauce

½ a small cabbage

½ cup of chicken stock

½teaspoon of crushed garlic

½ teaspoon of crushed ginger

Method

Clean and slice the spring onions, carrots, cabbage, pepper and string beans into thin strips 6-9cm (2-3 inches) in length.

Heat the sesame oil in a saucepan. Add the garlic and ginger and fry for about ½ minute. Stir in the chicken stock, soy sauce, brown sugar, lemon juice and a pinch of pepper and a dash of tobasco and bring to the boil. Mix in the cornflour and wine/sherry, and simmer for another ½ minute. Turn off the heat.

Heat a tablespoon of olive oil in a wok. Add the sliced spring onions, carrots, cabbage, pepper and sting beans and stir fry. Add the bean sprouts and stir until they begin to soften. Add the sauce from the saucepan. Bring to the boil and serve.

Cheats

You can use any meat, fish or vegetables in a stir fry, so use anything that you like.

Many shops sell pre-prepared packs of stir fry vegetables. These shops will also sell packets and jars of pour over stir fry sauce. This means that a stir fry meal can be made in a matter of minutes - far quicker than microwave cooking!

Fish with parsley sauce

(Contains: omega3, antioxidants, selenium, B vitamins and folic acid, vitamin B6, potassium)

Ingredients

2 large fillets of skinless white fish
½ a head of broccoli
3 tablespoons of frozen peas
800m I skimmed milk
40g plain flour
40g butter
4 tablespoons of chopped fresh parsley
Pepper
10-15 new potatoes

Method

Place the fish in a large frying pan and half-fill with water. Bring to the boil and simmer for 20 minutes. Rinse and cut (no need to peel) the new potatoes in halves and place in a saucepan of water. Bring to the boil and simmer gently for 10 minutes. Add the broccoli, bring to the boil and simmer for 5 minutes. Add the peas, bring to the boil and simmer for 5 minutes.

Melt the butter into a saucepan on a low heat. Stir in the flour and cook for 2 minutes. Remove from the heat and stir in the milk a little at a time (stir continuously to avoid lumps). Bring to the boil and simmer for 5 minutes. Remove from the heat and stir in the parsley and add pepper to taste.

Remove the fish from the pan and drain off any excess water.

Strain the potatoes, broccoli and peas. Serve on 2 plates and pour over the parsley sauce.

Cheats
Most shops sell jars of parsley sauce or cartons of sauce mix to which you add either milk or water.
You can use any vegetables you like.

Stew
(Contains: antioxidants, B vitamins and folic acid, vitamin B6, potassium, zinc)

Ingredients

  1 small swede (diced)
  1 tbsp chopped thyme
  1½kg stewing beef (diced)
  15 button mushrooms
  2 parsnips (diced)
  2 tbsp chopped parsley
  3 carrots (diced)
  3 onions (quartered)
  425ml chicken or beef stock
  425ml red wine
  Olive oil
  Salt and black pepper

Method

Brown the beef in the olive oil in a hot casserole or heavy saucepan.

Remove the meat and toss in the onions, mushrooms, parsnips, swede and carrots, one ingredient at a time, seasoning each time.

Place these back in the casserole, along with the parsley and thyme.

Cover with red wine and stock and simmer for one hour or until the meat and vegetables are cooked.

Cheats

For a small quantity of stew, it may be easier to use a packet of frozen casserole or stewing vegetables.
It may be easier to buy a packet or jar of casserole mix rather than using the wine and stock.

Any meat can be used, or you can simply make a vegetable stew.

Taking it further

The recipes above are useful because it is hard to make mistakes, and they allow you to vary the ingredients to suit your personal tastes. They all count as fast food, and they all use healthy ingredients.

Having tried these out, you may want to look for other recipes. With growing concern to promote healthy eating, you can now find recipes for healthy meals anywhere you choose to look in newspapers and magazines, on the Internet – YouTube is a particularly good source of recipes as it allows you to watch (and pause and rewind) the way a meal is prepared. You can also buy recipe books from all good bookshops.

Life Surfing

Food for Mood

Healthy eating is not as difficult or as time consuming as you may have been led to believe. Nor is it something that only well-off people are able to afford. Indeed, healthy eating is often cost effective eating too.

The barriers preventing healthy eating for people with mental health problems fall into two categories:

- o Food poverty barriers
- o Mental health barriers

Importantly, these can be overcome with a little patience and forward planning. The important thing is not to set yourself up to fail by trying to change radically overnight what you eat or the way you shop for, store and prepare food.

Often the meals we are already eating can be made healthier simply by tweaking the recipe - perhaps adding some fresh ingredients instead of processed ones. With a bit of forethought and some menu planning, you can begin to substitute healthy meals for less healthy ones.

Taking care to eat regular meals - especially breakfast – and finding daytime activities to prevent eating for comfort or to alleviate boredom are also worth doing.

One reason why people experiencing mental health problems give up on healthy eating is that it seldom delivers an immediate feel-good hit in the way that sugary foods and chocolate often do. However, while these quick-fix foods may make you feel good briefly, their long-term effect is to leave you feeling less well. In contrast, over time eating healthily will gradually improve your sense of wellbeing.

Unfortunately, nobody can promise that eating healthily alone will bring about recovery. For most people who have recovered from mental illness, it is a combination of factors such as getting the right medication, psychological therapies, physical activity, "sleep hygiene", social connection, economic activity and the recovery of hope that come together to promote recovery.

Nevertheless, eating healthily is an important factor in recovery for a large number of people. Moreover, a poor or deteriorating diet is likely to result in worsening health that, in turn, will exacerbate mental illness.

So there is every reason to eat healthily as an important step that you can take as part of your recovery. It won't hurt you, and it might just be the thing that kick-starts your progress towards recovery.

About Life Surfing

Life Surfing is a not-for-profit Community Interest Company that was established to provide a coaching, mentoring and training approach for people experiencing common life problems that can cause stress, anxiety and depression.

Our mission is to help people learn to cope with life without the need to call on over-stretched NHS services that are better deployed to help people with severe mental illness.

Over the years we have found that there is a huge amount that people can do to develop their personal resources and to foster their own wellbeing. In most cases, the real need is for encouragement, support, knowledge and skills.

This is what Life Surfing offers.

We have developed a range of services – one-to-one coaching, training workshops, mentoring groups and a range of publications - to give you the knowledge, skills and motivation needed to address life's issues and overcome stress-related problems in a healthy way, and to promote your long-term personal wellbeing.

For further information, please visit the Life Surfing website:

www.life-surfing.com
info@life-surfing.com

Or you can contact us on: 0300 321 4514 / 07922 537 646

Life Surfing
Box 124, R&R Consulting Centre
41 St. Isan Road
Heath
Cardiff CF14 4LW

Life Surfing is a community interest company limited by guarantee (07399335) registered in England and Wales

www.ingramcontent.com/pod-product-compliance
Lightning Source LLC
Chambersburg PA
CBHW070809290526
45795CB00002B/669